BELIEVE IN YOUR SELF

BOOST YOUR SELF-ESTEEM AND FEEL GOOD IN THE SKIN YOU'RE IN

Jasmin Kirkbride

BELIEVE IN YOURSELF

Text by Jasmin Kirkbride

Vie Books is an imprint of Summersdale Publishers Ltd

Summersdale Publishers Ltd
46 West Street
Chichester
West Sussex
PO19 1RP
UK

www.summersdale.com

Printed and bound in the Czech Republic

ISBN: 978-1-84953-949-4

Substantial discounts on bulk quantities of Summersdale books are available to corporations, professional associations and other organisations. For details contact Nicky Douglas by telephone: +44 (0) 1243 756902, fax: +44 (0) 1243 786300 or email: nicky@summersdale.com.

To..

From..

INTRODUCTION

TAKING THE FIRST STEPS

When I believe in myself, the whole world blooms for me.

Believing in yourself is so often easier said than done. Even if it's not a constant problem, some days you might just feel down on yourself. Perhaps you doubt you're good enough, or clever enough, or attractive enough – and scrolling through your social-media feeds definitely isn't helping!

This book is here to help you turn that negative spiral around so you can feel confident in the skin you're in. These tips and tricks aren't overnight solutions, but they will show you how to become happier and more confident by teaching you exactly how to be yourself and love yourself.

A journey of a thousand miles begins with a single step.

Lao Tzu

PART ONE

SELF-ESTEEM

I have more potential for goodness
than I can possibly imagine.

Self-esteem is the way that you think about yourself and how these thoughts make you feel and behave. Your opinions about what sort of person you are, your abilities, your place in the world and what your future looks like all affect your self-esteem. Low self-esteem can prevent you living life to the full if it makes you feel nervous in social situations, if it means you avoid challenges or stops you from trying new things. Feeling bad about yourself much of the time is enough to make anyone unhappy. The good news is that you can boost your self-esteem! This book shows you how.

**Believe in yourself…
Know that there is
something inside you
that is greater than
any obstacle.**

Christian D. Larson

WHO'S AFFECTED BY LOW SELF-ESTEEM?

A rough patch can happen to anyone – we all have days when we get out on the wrong side of the bed or we just don't seem to be able to do anything right. Low self-esteem is different: it affects people in the long-term and is caused by patterns of negative thinking. Sufferers from low self-esteem can pick up negative thought habits during childhood; or have these habits pushed on to them by family, friends, teachers or even the media; or they may develop them later in life for many reasons, including becoming self-conscious about their body image. Whatever the reason, the idea that they aren't good enough sticks with them.

I WILL LEARN TO APPRECIATE THE MOMENT.

I AM NOT WHAT HAS
HAPPENED TO ME.
I AM WHAT I CHOOSE
TO BECOME.

Carl Jung

DO I HAVE LOW SELF-ESTEEM?

Do you constantly tell yourself that you're going to fail at things, sometimes before you've even tried them? Do you automatically assume strangers will think you're silly? Do you only feel good when you've achieved something or made someone else happy? Are you hard on yourself? These are all signs of low self-esteem but it can be identified by different symptoms too. Other common signs include regularly feeling low, feeling worthless and choosing to avoid social situations.

Many people struggle with self-esteem at some point in their lives, but severe self-esteem issues can cause anxiety and depression. If you ever feel that everything is getting too much and you just can't deal with it, see your doctor and get extra help (there's more on this at the end of the book).

I AM NOT TRYING TO CHANGE MYSELF. I AM TRYING TO CHANGE THE WAY I THINK ABOUT MYSELF.

LEARN TO LOVE YOURSELF

Be nice to yourself! By practising kindness towards yourself, you can throw out old thinking patterns which drag you down and build up new habits that help you feel more positive day by day. Every single person is unique but there are some helpful trends, so read on to match yourself to one of the common types of self-esteem to understand yourself better – and discover what *you* can do to boost *your* self-belief!

IF I LEARN TO
LOVE MYSELF
EVERY DAY,
THE TIME WILL
COME WHEN I
FORGET THAT I
EVER DOUBTED
MY WORTH.

You yourself, as much as anybody in the entire universe, deserve your love and affection.

Buddha

SECURE HIGH SELF-ESTEEM

If you have secure high self-esteem, you have a relatively objective view of yourself – the way you see yourself and the way the world sees you are quite similar. You tend to be confident in your decisions and self-worth, and don't feel threatened if you need to argue your opinions. You're a good judge of when you've done the right thing and when you need to apologise. You're sensitive to others but know when to prioritise yourself – make sure that you don't ever lose sight of this!

I have faith in myself. I can do anything I set my mind to.

DEFENSIVE HIGH SELF-ESTEEM

If you think highly of yourself but aren't confident about it – so you feel vulnerable to criticism – you may have defensive high self-esteem. This means that while you may appear confident at first, you tend to become grumpy or upset if you get something wrong and someone calls you out on it or says something bad about you. Remember that you're only human and that everyone makes mistakes!

LETTING GO OF SOMETHING TAKES AS MUCH COURAGE AS FIGHTING AGAINST IT.

I am more awesome
than I know.

LOW SELF-ESTEEM

If you have low self-esteem, you often have negative thoughts about yourself, or only think well of yourself in certain conditions, which can make you very unhappy. You focus on your slip-ups instead of your achievements, blame yourself when things go wrong and are constantly questioning your worth. If this sounds like you, remember to think positive and stay positive!

WORTHINESS-BASED SELF-ESTEEM

Those who have worthiness-based self-esteem have relatively high self-esteem but it relies on other people respecting and liking them. Does this sound like you? If so, be aware of its influence on you in the long run, as you might feel pressured to live life according to your family's or friends' ideas of what's best for you. You might feel a strong desire to make other people happy even if that doesn't make *you* happy. Just be careful not to make too many sacrifices to please other people!

Accepting myself is more important than acceptance from anyone else.

COMPETENCE-BASED SELF-ESTEEM

High achievers find self-worth through racking up successes. You might well be the one getting excellent grades and good jobs or winning awards. Like those with worthiness-based self-esteem, you have high self-esteem but it's easily toppled because you only have high self-esteem if you're being successful. You can be highly critical of yourself even if you get the littlest thing wrong. Try not to be your own worst critic – don't beat yourself up!

MY **ACHIEVEMENTS** DO NOT MAKE ME WHO I AM; THEY ARE A **SIDE EFFECT** OF WHO I AM.

PART TWO

BOOSTING SELF-ESTEEM

When change seems daunting, just focus on putting one foot in front of the other.

There are lots of ways to boost self-esteem, and most of them are quite simple even if they may not always feel easy. By practising positivity and taking these practical steps in your everyday life, you can beat the low-self-esteem blues and enjoy your life to the full.

FACE YOUR ANXIETY
AND DO IT ANYWAY

There's a difference between fear and anxiety. Fears occur in life-threatening situations, such as seeing a car coming when you're crossing the road. Anxieties are things that worry you but don't objectively threaten your well-being, such as social anxiety and phobias.

A lot of people with low self-esteem experience anxieties and they're more likely to experience social anxiety, which makes events like hanging out with friends and going to parties seem scary. The natural reaction to anxiety is to try to avoid the situation, but this tactic is unhelpful in the long run. By avoiding the situation, you give credit to the idea that your anxiety is real and you prevent yourself from learning how to deal with it. Rather than avoiding the things that worry you, face them head-on. Get up, get out there and learn to overcome your anxieties

WHEN I FEEL AFRAID, I WILL REMEMBER THAT THE WORLD IS NOT WAITING TO JUDGE ME.

COURAGE IS NOT THE ABSENCE OF FEAR, BUT RATHER THE JUDGEMENT THAT SOMETHING ELSE IS MORE IMPORTANT THAN FEAR.

Meg Cabot

You are braver than you believe, stronger than you seem, and smarter than you think.

A. A. Milne

Start where you are. Use what you have. Do what you can.

Arthur Ashe

SET YOURSELF GOALS

Feeling listless or isolated? Don't know where you're heading or what to do with yourself? Then it's time to set some goals! Aim to fit your goals in with the rest of your life and be clear exactly what you want to accomplish. Goals like 'worry less' are a bit vague and may make you more anxious. 'Learn how to cook pasta' or 'be able to do ten push-ups in a row' are more focused goals with a definite end point, so you'll feel a satisfying sense of achievement when you hit your target. As your achievements turn into larger ones, such as becoming a fantastic all-round cook or becoming fitter, you'll find yourself feeling more confident in your abilities and skills.

GET A HOBBY OR
JOIN A CLUB

If you've never had a hobby before, now is the time to pick one up. If you have a hobby, make sure you give yourself plenty of time to indulge in it. It could be anything – painting, playing an instrument, knitting – but the important bit is that you love doing it and that it makes you happy. Enjoy this 'me time'!

Picking up a hobby, joining a club or taking a class will help you gain a sense of achievement, but it will also give you a social context. Being part of a club allows you to meet people but the pressure is off because everyone's focused on a common activity. For full benefits, choose something you really enjoy doing and go regularly.

I WILL REJOICE IN THE SMALL THINGS. A LITTLE SOMETHING EACH DAY BUILDS A BIG SOMETHING IN A YEAR.

YOU BECOME WHAT YOU DO, SO I WILL DO SOMETHING I LOVE.

WORK IT OUT

A job, whether it's paid or voluntary work, can help you feel more assured about your abilities and value. As with joining a club, work gives you a social context, a place to be and people to hang out with. It also provides you with a strong sense of purpose and achievement, which can be very beneficial in increasing self-esteem.

Always ensure that you keep a good balance between your work and home life though. While work is important, so is downtime!

BOOST YOUR BODY LANGUAGE

The way we hold ourselves really affects how we feel. Many people with low self-esteem tend to hunch over, as if closing themselves off or hiding themselves away, and this body language doesn't send out the most positive message to the world.

Consciously open up and relax your body. Breathe deep into your belly, and on the out-breath let go of any tension in your body. Release your shoulders and roll them back and down so that you're standing tall. By consciously being more confident in your posture, you appear more confident to the outside world; you'll soon find confidence growing within yourself.

I WILL GIVE
MYSELF
PURPOSE, AND
CONFIDENCE
WILL COME.

Every time I fall, I will get back up and stand taller than I was before.

When you have confidence, you can have a lot of fun.

Joe Namath

EXPRESS YOURSELF

Aim to speak positively and assertively. Being assertive isn't about being like a bull in a china shop; it's about respecting others' needs and feelings – and expecting the same from them towards you.

To express your feelings, wait until you've processed the situation, then explain what's going on to the others involved. When you talk about yourself, use the first person ('I feel… I think… When you do this to me…') as this can help you explain things without feeling angry or nervous.

Being assertive isn't always easy, even for people with high self-esteem, but you can do it – just keep trying. Practise with yourself in the mirror and you'll be asserting your opinions in no time.

MY FEELINGS AND MY THOUGHTS ARE AS LEGITIMATE AND IMPORTANT AS EVERYONE ELSE'S. I WILL NOT BE AFRAID TO EXPRESS THEM.

**WITHOUT 'YES',
I CANNOT
WELCOME
OPPORTUNITY.
WITHOUT 'NO',
I CANNOT
STAND UP FOR
MY NEEDS.
WITH BOTH,
I CAN LIVE A
BALANCED LIFE.**

A 'NO' IS AS GOOD AS A 'YES'

A key part of being assertive and being able to express your needs is learning to say 'no'. A lot of people find that saying 'no' brings them out in a cold sweat, but it can be a useful, positive word. By saying 'yes' all the time, you may find yourself in undesirable situations, becoming resentful and upset, with way too much on your plate.

Saying 'no' – with a nice explanation of why not, if it's appropriate – doesn't harm relationships for the most part, but it does allow you to express what you need. In fact, people may trust you more, because they'll understand that you're fully committed to the things you do say 'yes' to. Plus, by giving yourself what you need, you'll become happier and less stressed!

STOP COMPARING YOURSELF

The comparison game can just as easily happen offline as online. Remember that life is not a race to achieve or experience milestone events first. Everybody has their own path and you should travel along yours in a way that's meaningful to you. Other people's successes are not your failings. Don't waste your time on jealousy – everything you are and everything that you are not is what makes you unique.

We need to learn to love ourselves first, in all our glory and imperfections.

John Lennon

WHY WOULD I TRY TO BE SOMEBODY ELSE**, WHEN I AM SO** AMAZING**?**

PART THREE

CONTROLLING NEGATIVE THOUGHTS

Positivity is what happens
when you use your imagination
for the power of good.

We all have inner voices telling us things about ourselves. For people with low self-esteem, these voices tend to speak negatively whether or not those things are true. By turning these negative thoughts into positive ones, you can transform the way you feel about yourself.

THIS VERY MOMENT
IS A SEED FROM
WHICH THE FLOWERS
OF TOMORROW'S
HAPPINESS GROW.

Margaret Lindsay

IDENTIFY NEGATIVE THOUGHTS

The first step in changing negative thought patterns is to identify what they are. Do you always think you'll fail? Or that you're ugly? Or that you say stupid things whenever you open your mouth? Or are you afraid what other people think about you?

Sit down in a quiet space with a few hours to yourself and write down what your inner voices are saying. What negative thoughts crop up again and again? Then write down positive things that have happened which challenge your self-doubts and you'll soon come to realise that your worst thoughts aren't true!

Good things are going to happen to me, even if I can't see it yet.

ONCE I IDENTIFY THE **BEGINNING,** I CAN SEE HOW FAR I'VE COME.

UNDERSTAND WHERE NEGATIVE THOUGHTS COME FROM

It might help to figure out where your negative thoughts originate from, or when they started. Was it when you didn't pass that exam? Or when you had an outbreak of acne? Was it when you moved house?

Working out where your negative thoughts came from can really help you to understand your thought processes, and you can begin to move on and build up more positive thoughts instead. Stop dwelling on what's over and done with, and instead of focusing on negative aspects of past events, focus on the positive things you've learnt from them – things which will help you deal with future challenges.

LET GO OF NEGATIVE THOUGHTS

When you're trying to change the way you think, it's common to try to push the bad thoughts away, to shove them out of your mind completely. Instead of resisting them, relax into your thoughts and let them move *through* your mind.

By pushing negativity away, you're actually engaging with the thought and are likely to follow it up and keep thinking about it. It's much more effective to stand back and observe your negative thoughts, almost as if they belong to someone else, and let them pass by like clouds in the sky. Don't cling or push; just let them float past, then move on to nicer things.

I will allow each
situation to be what it
is instead of what I am
worried it might be.

WHEN I'M FEELING LOW, I WILL WRITE OUT THE BAD TO MAKE ROOM FOR THE GOOD.

WRITE IT OUT

For some people, recognising negative thoughts can be challenging. If you're finding it hard, try writing a diary. Start to keep an honest, private journal and read back over it every week or so, looking out for the recurring thoughts that made you feel sad or discouraged. These might include blaming yourself, feeling ashamed about things that aren't your fault, or making something worse in your head than it actually was.

Writing everything down will help you to put it into perspective. Aim to record at least one positive thing every day, as well as whatever you're feeling, then build this number up over time. Your diary will help you focus on the good stuff.

MAKE A
FEEL-GOOD LIST

Just as you wrote down the bad things you think about yourself, now it's time to write down all the good stuff! Make a list of the things you like about your personality and your body. Write down what you're good at and the compliments people have given you. Keep at it until you have at least ten things on your list, and add to it over time. Now you don't just have a list of the negative thoughts to overcome – you've got lots of awesome things to focus on as well!

THE MORE
I FOCUS ON
THE POSITIVE,
THE EASIER IT
BECOMES.

ONE POSITIVE THOUGHT GIVES BIRTH TO TWO MORE.

THINK POSITIVE

One of the most helpful treatments for anxiety and self-esteem issues is Cognitive Behavioural Therapy (CBT). It's actually not as tricky as it sounds, and a lot of it is about getting into the habit of thinking nice or neutral things rather than the negative ones you might be used to.

When your worst thoughts strike, turn your inner voice around and make it tell you the positive, not the negative. Tell yourself you can do it and that everything will be OK. Use your past experience to build an argument against your negative thoughts. For example, if you're convinced that nobody likes you, remember who called you on your birthday, an upcoming event you've been invited to or the interesting conversation you had with a friend yesterday.

Learning to think positively can be hard, but keep at it and soon you won't even notice you're doing it. You'll be well on the way to loving yourself and feeling great about being you!

BELIEVE YOU CAN AND YOU'RE HALFWAY THERE.

THEODORE ROOSEVELT

I will feel love for myself.

COMPASSION

Compassion is very important in turning the self-esteem boat around, but it can be challenging because it involves learning to love yourself *unconditionally*. Compassion is love, but it's not romantic and has no strings attached. It's a universal feeling of acceptance towards everything – most importantly, in this case, yourself.

Being compassionate towards yourself doesn't mean being selfish. Selfishness comes from a place of emptiness and need, but self-love comes from a place of kindness and understanding. Take the pressure off, give yourself a break and be kind towards yourself and your body, and see how quickly you start feeling better.

**To love oneself
is the beginning of a
lifelong romance.**

Oscar Wilde

EVEN IF I CAN'T BE **POSITIVE** ALL THE TIME, I WILL MAKE **HAPPINESS** A HABIT.

GO EASY ON YOUR BRAIN

Positive thinking is like a muscle that you have to exercise – you're training your brain to think differently. Retraining doesn't happen overnight, and getting rid of negative thoughts takes time and practice, so if you slip up be gentle with yourself. Don't give yourself a hard time because that's just another negative thought pattern. Instead, give yourself a mental cuddle, forgive yourself and move on. Positivity starts right here and right now.

START BY DOING WHAT'S NECESSARY; THEN DO WHAT'S POSSIBLE; AND SUDDENLY YOU ARE DOING THE IMPOSSIBLE.

Francis of Assisi

PART FOUR

SOCIAL MEDIA AND SELF-ESTEEM

Don't let other people
define who you are.

Social media plays a huge role in our lives and self-esteem nowadays. Whether you're a Twitter fanatic or a Reddit addict, the chances are you've got a profile out there somewhere. Social media is a great way to connect with people but it's not always easy on self-esteem. Instagram, Facebook, Vine, Snapchat, likes, friends, notifications – it can be overwhelming! So here are a few tips to help you knock social-media anxiety on the head.

Attitude is a little thing that makes a big difference.

Winston Churchill

THE COMPARISON GAME

Having an online window into other people's lives might make you feel more in touch with them, but it doesn't necessarily make you feel good about yourself. It's very tempting to compare ourselves to others on social media, and because people tend to post only the best stuff about their lives online, we can end up feeling glum and inadequate at the end of a browsing session.

But there are things you can do to stop the shame spiral. When you feel that you're getting sucked into the comparison game, remind yourself of a recent happy memory or of an event you're looking forward to, and remind yourself that *your* life is awesome. Stop following or visiting the profiles of people who you know will make you feel bad. Instead, regularly clear out your newsfeed to ensure that you're following pages with fun and inspiring posts that you actually enjoy.

REJOICING IN OTHER PEOPLE DOESN'T MEAN BRINGING MYSELF DOWN. I AM JUST AS WONDERFUL AS EVERYONE ELSE.

Happiness is a journey, not a destination.

Souza

FEAR OF MISSING OUT (FOMO)

You could be at home happily watching your way through a few episodes of a TV programme or reading a book, when a photo of some friends at a party pops up on your newsfeed. Your contented bubble has suddenly disappeared. Now you feel lonely and inadequate. Why is everyone else having more fun than you? And why didn't they invite you along? We've all felt it – FOMO is a beast. It can make us agree to do things we don't really want to, just because we're worried we're going to miss out on something or not be included in the selfies that would make us look cool online. If you feel a wave of FOMO coming on, stop. Instead, choose to boost your self-esteem by giving yourself what you need. Choose to do things because you genuinely want to, not because you think they'll look good for your image or your new profile picture.

I WILL DO WHAT I LOVE, AND LOVE WHAT I DO.

Beauty begins the moment you decide to be yourself.

Coco Chanel

IGNORE IMPOSSIBLE STANDARDS

Ever seen a photo of someone online then wanted to cover yourself up because you think you don't look as good as them? You're not the only one. The unrealistic expectations of the media and fashion industry have a lot to answer for, including rising rates of eating disorders and social anxiety, which are starting at increasingly younger ages.

If you feel yourself getting down, remind yourself that these standards are impossible and that many images in the mainstream media have been edited. The 'perfect' photos in adverts and magazines encourage many of us to enhance photos before posting them online when we're already perfect just the way we are in real life.

Still feel the self-hate coming on? Take a second to close your eyes, breathe and really reach out to your body with your mind. Give yourself a hug and tell yourself, in your head or out loud, that you're beautiful. Because – trust me – you are.

I will not worry about
what other people think.
I will be a sunflower
amongst daisies.

TO BE **YOURSELF**
IN A WORLD THAT
IS CONSTANTLY
TRYING TO
MAKE YOU
SOMETHING ELSE
IS THE **GREATEST**
ACCOMPLISHMENT.

DEAL WITH PEER PRESSURE

We're told that we should be doing lots of things – smoking or having sex – to make ourselves 'cool' and social media intensifies this peer pressure. A lot of it is nonsense but, even so, it can be hard to ignore. Perhaps it seems that 'everyone' is doing these things, but if they're not up your street then the best thing you can do is to remain true to yourself. Don't do something unless you're ready and you truly want to do it. Standing out like this takes bravery and may make you feel anxious or insecure, especially if you have low self-esteem, but sticking to your guns about what's right for you is a crucial step in being kind to yourself.

'No' is a legitimate word online and in the real world. If you're ever in a situation where you're finding it hard to stand up to peer pressure, remind yourself that what *you* want and need is valid and important.

STOP COUNTING LIKES

A lot of people seem to think that your worth as a human being and a friend is based on how many likes you get, how many messages you receive in a day and how many followers you have. This is absolutely not true. For starters, social media edits what appears in your newsfeeds, so other people might not even see your posts at all – they may not be online when you post. Enjoy likes when they happen, but don't fret if you don't get loads, just move on and remember that it's not personal.

I can change the world, but the world doesn't have to change me.

You are your own judge. The verdict is up to you.

Astrid Alauda

QUALITY, NOT QUANTITY

Another social media contest that dents your self-esteem is comparing numbers of friends and followers. Some people may have more than you; other people may have fewer. When it comes to friends, the secret is quality, not quantity.

If you find yourself getting wound up by the online numbers game, take a step back. Meet up with someone face-to-face and do something fun and relaxing. Getting a real-life hug from three people will boost your brain's happy sensors more than getting ten new followers!

ONE STAR SHINES
BRIGHTER THAN
A THOUSAND
CANDLES.

IF YOU WANT TO IMPROVE YOUR SELF-WORTH, STOP GIVING OTHER PEOPLE THE CALCULATOR.

TIM FARGO

CYBERBULLYING

Cyberbullying can seriously damage your self-esteem, turning social media from a fun, friendly tool into a world of worry and distress.

If you experience online bullying, the first thing to do is to take a step back from your screens and devices. Close your eyes and breathe deeply into your stomach until the initial stress has gone away. Try to talk it out with the person involved, but if they don't want to talk, or things get worse, feel free to block them or tell someone who is in a position to help.

Don't put up with people treating you badly online or in real life. Part of the process of building up your self-esteem is understanding that you don't deserve to be treated badly and knowing you can do something about it.

Turn my screen off; turn my life on.

TAKE TIME OUT

Social media is addictive. Fact. Getting likes and notifications lights up those juicy reward centres in your brain, making you crave them, so you check your accounts again and again throughout the day. These reward centres are also what make you feel sad when you don't get any likes or any comments.

What's more, repeatedly logging into Facebook and other websites may make you feel like you're getting less interaction than you really are, and this can inflict a bad dose of self-doubt.

The advice on this is simple: log in less, and limit the amount of time you spend on social media when you do use it. Remember to engage with the real, offline world!

PART FIVE

MINDFULNESS

I will live my day being aware of its
connection to my whole life.

Let's be honest: sitting with your thoughts can be pretty daunting if you've got an inner voice that just won't shut up. However, this can be exactly what you need to do to increase your self-esteem. Mindfulness teaches your brain to think clearly and positively, to overcome the negative thoughts and welcome the good ones.

There are lots of ways to practise mindfulness. Here are several methods that are particularly good for boosting self-esteem. Aim to 'do' a little bit of mindfulness every day, even if it's only ten minutes, because the more you practise, the more natural it will become.

I was always looking outside myself for strength and confidence but it comes from within.

Anna Freud

WITH THE NEW
DAY COMES NEW
STRENGTH AND
NEW THOUGHTS.

Eleanor Roosevelt

NO JUDGEMENT

Make a deal with yourself before you start this practice that whatever you find in your head, you'll meet it with love and kindness. Turn all your screens off, put your phone on silent and go to a quiet place where you can sit comfortably. Relax your eyelids, straighten your back without straining, and put your hands in your lap or on your knees. Breathe into your belly, feeling your ribs expand outwards, and touch base with your body. How are you feeling right now?

After a few moments, spread your senses outwards, notice the sounds around you, the feel of the floor or seat beneath you. Just sit in the moment, let your mind hang loose and let your thoughts pass through you without judgement. This practice isn't about trying to make the moment 'perfect' – it's about appreciating the present moment. Don't strain to get it 'right', just let everything *be* in a gentle space.

I WILL LISTEN TO MY BODY, TAKE CARE OF IT AND LOVE IT.

BODY SCAN

Thinking negative things about yourself can be a difficult habit to break, but you can get back in touch with your brain and body, and trust them to be positive.

In a still, quiet space, sit comfortably or lie down. Breathe in deep and centre yourself. Relax. When you next breathe in, imagine you're breathing right into your toes. As you breathe out, consciously relax your toes and imagine that you're breathing out all the negativity. Repeat this all the way up your body, relaxing each part as you go.

When you reach the top of your head, turn your attention inwards to your mind. As in previous exercises, watch your thoughts like they're clouds in the sky, without either grasping at them or pushing them away. Just breathe around your thoughts as they pass through you.

SEE THE LIGHT!

Visualisation is a great technique for building more positivity in your life. Having a regular visualisation practice gives you a safe place to go when your thoughts turn mean. While you're doing one of the mindfulness exercises in this book, begin to imagine your body slowly filling with a soft, golden light. Start at your heart and let the light seep outwards in your mind, until it fills every part of you, right down to your fingers and toes. The light should feel kind, warm and gentle. Once you've filled yourself with it, imagine the light starting to seep out of your skin, filling the room, the house, the town – maybe even the world!

I WILL ALLOW
THE WORLD
TO FILL ME
WITH LOVE,
AND LOVE IT
IN RETURN.

I WILL ALLOW MYSELF TO BECOME THE PERSON I WANT TO BE.

PICTURE YOUR FUTURE SELF

People suffering low self-esteem often see difficult or lonely futures for themselves. Thinking your future will be bad doesn't exactly make you want to jump up and down in your present. But the great thing is that the future hasn't happened yet, so you can turn it into whatever you want it to be! Sitting in a quiet place, get into a mindful headspace and focus on your breath. Picture your future self as someone who's happy and fulfilled. You can add in specifics to do with your goals and dreams, like your dream job or excellent exam results. The most important thing is to picture this future you as confident and surrounded by love. By picturing it clearly, you can make it happen.

It is in
our darkest
moments that
we must focus
to see the light.

Buddha

PART SIX

SLEEPING

I will let go of today. Tomorrow will be
a brand new start.

On average, you need about eight hours' sleep a night, and having at least a couple of those before midnight is ideal. Sleep is key to helping your body and mind reset; not getting enough sleep can make you think more negatively because your body is stressed. When your mind keeps ticking and your inner voices are giving you a hard time, it can be difficult to stop tossing and turning, so here are some tricks to help you get off to the land of nod.

I believe that tomorrow is another day and I believe in miracles.

Audrey Hepburn

We are all of us stars, and we deserve to twinkle.

Marilyn Monroe

BEDTIME ROUTINE

Yes, bedtime routines are for grown-ups too! Having a set routine before bed trains your mind and body to expect bedtime and be ready for it by the time you get there.

Try to get to bed around the same time every night – making exceptions for parties, of course! Start preparing for bed by turning off all your screens and sounds. Then brush your teeth, wash your face, adding in a bath or shower if you want. Tuck yourself up in bed and take some time to unwind. Maybe you want to read a book or perhaps this is the time you write in your diary; just make sure you pick a non-digital activity. After half an hour, or when you start to get drowsy, close your book or diary, turn the light off and settle down.

It can take a while for the body to get used to a new routine, so keep at it and soon you'll be getting to sleep in no time.

TURN OFF THE SCREENS

This is a key tip: stay away from screens for at least an hour before bed. The blue light given out by LED and TV screens tricks your brain into thinking it's still daytime and that you aren't sleepy yet. Actually, you might be exhausted, but you wouldn't realise until you stopped looking at the screen. This artificial light makes your brain more active in general, meaning it takes you longer to wind down once you do get to bed.

If you don't want to switch off completely, there are apps that gradually dim your device's screen with a red tint to counter the blue light. But to really allow your brain to really get ready for sleep, just turn off the tech!

I WILL NOT BE AFRAID OF LETTING MYSELF REFUEL, RESET AND SLEEP.

WHETHER I HAVE **CONTROL** OR NOT, I WILL **TRUST** THAT THINGS WILL **WORK OUT.**

IS YOUR BODY KEEPING YOU UP?

Your body being in a still, relaxed state is a huge part of getting to sleep. Be careful not to eat too close to bedtime as a full stomach and digestion disrupt your sleep, but make sure you're not hungry either. Avoid sugary or caffeinated drinks, which will keep you awake; instead a cup of herbal tea, chamomile for instance, can be very comforting around bedtime. Taking long naps in the afternoon or early evening will prevent your body from wanting to fall asleep later on. If you need to rest, take a quick power nap, not too late in the day. Exercising during the day helps get your body in a state of sleep-readiness by wearing it out, so get up off that chair and out into the world for a bit.

I will rest both my mind and my body.

Don't seek, don't search, don't ask... relax. If you relax, it comes.

Osho

THINK ABOUT SLEEP POSITIVELY

When sleep is evading us, it can seem like a faraway destination that's difficult to reach. But when you're fully relaxed, sleep is a very natural state for your body to fall into and you don't have to work for it. In fact, the more you struggle to sleep, the more your body will tense and your mind will worry. Let go of trying to get to sleep and trust that your body knows how to get there – it always does eventually.

BEDTIME IS THE CHANCE FOR ME TO NOT WORRY ABOUT ANYTHING – NOT EVEN ABOUT GETTING TO SLEEP!

PART SEVEN

RELAXATION

I won't judge the day before it's begun. Awesome things can happen if I open my mind to the possibility that they exist.

An important part of building more positivity into your life is winding down and chilling out. When you relax, your body lets go of its stress and tension, helping you become happier. The happier you are, the happier your thoughts will be!

RELEASE YOUR STRUGGLE, LET GO OF YOUR MIND, THROW AWAY YOUR CONCERNS, AND RELAX INTO THE WORLD.

DAN MILLMAN

ACUPRESSURE

There are pressure points all over your body which have different effects when you stimulate them. The art of acupressure is knowing how to use these pressure points and applying this to your everyday life.

There are lots of ways to use acupressure to help you feel more relaxed, but some of the easiest pressure points to find are on your temples and in your hands. These are simple, in-the-moment exercises you can do anywhere.

To ease tension, find the flat parts on either side of your head beside your eyes. Apply gentle pressure with two or three fingers, and rub in slow circles. Carry on for about two minutes, changing direction halfway through.

For relaxation, use the pressure points in your hands. Squeeze the fleshy, webbed bit of skin between your thumb and forefinger, getting as close to the place where the bones meet as you can. Hold for two minutes, then repeat on the other hand.

CRACK A SMILE

When you smile, the whole world looks better. Your body associates smiling with feeling good, so on a day-to-day level if you make an effort to smile more, the positivity will feed through to the rest of your life.

Even better is having a good belly laugh – it's like a smile on rocket fuel! Laughing actively lowers your body's stress levels and encourages your brain to release happy chemicals. If there's no one around to crack a joke with, try watching a funny video, listening to an amusing podcast or reading a laugh-out-loud book. You could even give a free laughter or laughter yoga class a try. Just make sure you giggle your socks off as often as possible!

I WILL BREAK
MY HABIT OF
NEGATIVE
THINKING
HOWEVER I CAN.

HE HAS ACHIEVED
SUCCESS WHO
HAS LIVED WELL,
LAUGHED OFTEN
AND LOVED MUCH.

Bessie Anderson Stanley

PUT ON SOME TUNES

Trying to escape a low-self-esteem spiral? Having trouble disconnecting from social media? Then crank up the tunes and blast the music! Listen to music that fits how you want to feel rather than how you do feel in the moment. Music can dramatically change your emotions, so go for something happy or relaxing. Dancing and singing along helps to get your body moving and put you in a positive frame of mind.

Life isn't about waiting for the storm to pass; it's about learning to dance in the rain.

Anonymous

When the chips are down, I will accept that I feel sad but I won't wallow in it. I will do something to shift the mood.

HAVE SOME GREEN TIME

Getting outside, away from concrete and into nature has a very positive effect on your mental state. Go somewhere you can feel the grass under your feet and the wind on your face; winter or summer, fresh air and green time do you so much good.

Whether you're at the beach or in a forest, take time to appreciate the little details – the sunshine through the leaves or the sound of the waves. Relax your walk to an amble, take the day as it comes and feel your worries being blown away.

I WILL TAKE TIME TO LIE IN THE SUNSHINE.

As soon as you trust yourself, you will know how to live.

Johann Wolfgang von Goethe

TAKE A BATH

A long, hot bath does wonders for the soul. The sensation of being in water and being able to totally relax allows your body to release all its tension. Adding in bubbles and lighting a few candles (safely away from your hair!) will give a sense of luxury. A decent bath is a real treat and an excellent way to care for yourself.

After a bath, your body takes 15–30 minutes to cool down. This cooling process is very effective at sending you off to sleep, so take this time to wind down and recoup. Dry off, wrap yourself in a warm blanket or duvet, curl up in a comfortable place and enjoy the moment.

POSITIVITY IS PHYSICAL AS WELL AS MENTAL. BY TREATING MY BODY, I'M TREATING MY MIND – AND THEY'LL BOTH BE GRATEFUL.

PART EIGHT

WELL-BEING

Building confidence isn't about
changing so I can like myself; it's about
loving myself so I can change.

Part of the process of boosting your self-esteem is realising that you can be beautiful and feel confident whatever you look like. You really can – there is no standard for 'beauty'. This section isn't about changing your body because you want to change the way you look. It's about altering what you eat and how you exercise to improve the way you feel and this is a very important distinction to make. Say something nice to yourself whenever you look in a mirror because you truly are worth it.

It's not the mountain we conquer, but ourselves.

Edmund Hillary

IF I DON'T
GIVE MY MIND
THE RIGHT FUEL,
IT CAN'T TRAVEL
TO THE STARS.

EAT HEALTHILY

The saying 'You are what you eat' is so true! When you don't feed your body the nutrition it needs, it panics and feels run down. This can make you sluggish, anxious, sad or cross – and it compromises the body's immune system, meaning that you're more likely to get sick or feel unwell.

Aim to eat at least your five a day of fruit and vegetables, with slow-burning carbohydrates like wholegrain rice or pasta on the side. Mix in some proteins – like nuts, meat, dairy, eggs and particularly fish, which is full of great, stress-busting nutrients. Ensure that all the right vitamins and minerals are included in your diet too (if in doubt, try some supplements to top you up). The antioxidant vitamins A, C and E will help combat the symptoms of stress. Vitamins D and B will boost your mood. Take care of your eating habits and you're well on your way to a happier body and a healthier mind.

THINGS TO AVOID

When we're feeling low, there can be a real temptation to binge-eat or, conversely, to not eat at all. Neither of these are good for fighting negative thoughts. Eating lots of saturated fat and sugary foods will give you crashes and make you feel lethargic, while keeping vital nutrients from your body will only make you feel lower.

Be careful what you drink too. Although caffeine may hype you up in the short-term, once it's worn off it can cause drowsiness and grumpiness, and will interrupt your natural sleeping patterns. Say no to booze, which is a depressant, and definitely keep your hands off drugs.

Coming off these types of food and drink can make you feel a bit rough in the first few days because they're all slightly addictive, but be disciplined and you'll soon notice a difference in the way you think and feel.

Exerting self-control over my diet isn't about starving myself; it's about eating better.

SOMETIMES, ALL I NEED TO LEVEL MYSELF OUT IS A GLASS OF WATER AND A HEALTHY SNACK.

STAY HYDRATED

Fruit juice and fizzy pop might taste great but they have a high sugar content. The best thing you can drink is pure water. Water is amazing for your body: it helps your skin stay healthy and pimple-free, it makes all your organs run smoothly, and it helps keep your brain nice and hydrated for thinking positively and staying focused. Water really is a miracle drink.

Non-caffeinated herbal teas can be very beneficial too and many have their own unique qualities. For example, chamomile is great for helping you sleep, while peppermint is good for calming the stomach. If you're missing coffee, ginger tea gives you a natural zing to keep you going throughout the day.

I don't think limits.

Usain Bolt

EXERCISE

Exercise isn't all about slimming down and toning up, though these can be pleasant side effects. It has lots of other benefits that are far more important if you have low self-esteem or lack confidence. For starters, exercise restores your ability to concentrate. It also releases one of your body's happy hormones, endorphins.

It doesn't have to be strenuous or difficult – exercise just means movement. A walk will do. Keep it fun by finding an exercise you love and teaming up with a friend to support each other. YouTube has loads of great free exercise videos if you want to connect to an online fitness community, or you could join a local sports club. Set aside two or three hour-long sessions per week to work out and do a little something to exercise every day, even if it's just a ten-minute walk down the road.

MOVE AND LIVE MINDFULLY

Some of the best exercises for boosting self-confidence are the ones which encourage you to consciously get in touch with your body. Gentle exercises like t'ai chi, yoga, Pilates and body balance all combine movement with mindfulness. The rhythmic breathing patterns align the body and mind, bringing you back down to earth, to the here and now, and focus your attention on linking your body and mind. What better way to help boost your positive vibes?

Look after yourself and treat your body as a temple. Do your nails, go for a run, attend to a daily skincare routine, stretch – find something which grounds you to your body and helps you appreciate it. Pay attention to your body and its needs, and you'll soon start to feel better about yourself. You are amazing just the way you are – all you have to do is appreciate and believe it.

A healthy relationship with my body will give me confidence!

PART NINE

TALKING AND FINDING HELP

If I'm feeling lonely, it's not because there's something wrong with me – it might just be that I haven't met the right people yet.

Talking about your low self-esteem might seem daunting, but the truth is that your friends and family love you and they want to help you become more positive towards yourself. Change can be tricky, and having someone there for you is a massive help.

Everyone discusses their problems differently, but whatever your style is, approach your problems gently. You can reveal as much or as little as you want to the other person – it's your call.

COURAGE IS NOT
HAVING THE
STRENGTH TO GO
ON – IT IS GOING ON
WHEN YOU DON'T
HAVE THE STRENGTH.

Napoléon Bonaparte

CREATE A SUPPORT NETWORK

Spend time with people who are nice to you and help you feel good about yourself. Not all friendships are necessarily good for you; in fact, some friendships can be toxic for self-esteem, especially if the so-called friends are highly critical. Focus your energy on people who are really rooting for you, and you'll soon find you're rooting for yourself too. While looking after yourself and your needs, practise kindness towards others too. If you're nice and supportive, hopefully people will be nice and supportive back – love does make the world go round, after all!

Talking to people you love and trust about your problems will help you to build up the support network you need to keep improving your self-esteem. Identify family or friends who you know you can rely on when times get tough. Once you start being open about your issues, you might well find that other people are going through similar things, which can be an incredibly sharing and supportive experience.

Walking with a friend in the dark is better than walking alone in the light.

Helen Keller

THE SPARK OF **HEALING** IS ALREADY **INSIDE** ME. I WILL FAN IT INTO **FLAMES.**

CONSIDER COUNSELLING

If it ever gets way too much and you feel like you can't cope, you can always seek counselling. The best first step is to go to your doctor and talk to them confidentially about what's going on in your life. They might recommend that you see a counsellor, or they may give you some medication to help.

If your situation is urgent and you can't wait to see the doctor there are some excellent helplines you can call. To find out more, visit:

www.mind.org.uk
www.samaritans.org
www.anxietyuk.org.uk
www.turn2me.org

THERE'S NOTHING SHAMEFUL ABOUT NEEDING A HELPING HAND. ASKING FOR HELP MEANS I AM NOT GIVING UP. I CAN MAKE IT!

CONCLUSION

MOVING FORWARD

I believe in myself. I've got this.

Even on your darkest days, practise trying to see the light. Be kind to yourself. Respect yourself. Embrace the relationship you have with your body and your mind. Don't get involved with worrying about what other people may or may not think, or about what may or may not happen. Enjoy the moment. Enjoy *your* life. Above all, keep going and keep learning to love yourself, and, one day soon, you won't even remember what it was like not to love the skin you're in.

In the depths of winter, I finally learned that there was in me an invincible summer.

Albert Camus

If you're interested in finding out more about our books, find us on Facebook at **Summersdale Publishers** and follow us on Twitter at **@Summersdale**.

www.summersdale.com